CW00417312

FEEL GOOD WEIGHT LOSS
FOR LIFE

THE SECRET OF HOW TO SUSTAINABLY LOSE
WEIGHT AND KEEP IT OFF FOR LIFE

KERRY JOHNSON

COPYRIGHT © KERRY JOHNSON 2020

All rights reserved. No part of this publication may be reproduced, stored in a retrieval system, or transmitted in any form or by any means electronic, mechanical recording or otherwise, without prior written permission of the author, except by a reviewer, who may quote brief passages in review.

The author nor the publisher is engaged in rendering health, medical, psychological, financial, legal, or other professional services to the individual reader. The ideas, procedures, and suggestions contained in this book are not intended as a substitute for consulting with your physician. Any use of the information in this book is at the reader's discretion. All matters regarding your health require medical supervision. Before starting any new eating or exercise regime always consult with your doctor first. Before you begin any healthcare program or change your lifestyle, you will consult with your physician or licensed healthcare practitioner to ensure that you are in good health and that examples contained in this book will not harm you. Neither the author nor the publisher shall be liable for any loss or damage allegedly arising from any information or suggestion in this book.

TO FAMILY

CONTENTS

INTRODUCTION

A ONE TRACK MIND

This is quite possibly one of the shortest books you'll ever read on weight loss and, ironically, much of it isn't about food or eating. You'll find no complicated explanations of how food is broken down by the body or the science of your appetite. You'll find no calorie counts or food lists and you won't find a single rule or guideline on how you should or shouldn't eat.

That is because eating is nothing more than a fundamental process needed to keep you alive. It is no different than breathing or drinking and I'm not about to suggest how you do these either. You are an amazingly intelligent person living in one of the most complex and evolved bodies known to science. You don't need to be told how to eat, no matter how much current culture has tried to convince you otherwise.

Every diet book, magazine, blog, website, app, group or social media site (to name but a few) I have ever tried have always told me that they're different. However, in one fundamental - and flawed - way, they are all the same. They are all about food and how to eat it, and I'm about to tell that's where it all goes wrong.

CHAPTER 1

THE IMPOSSIBILITY OF DIETING

Let me take you back to May 2019. Not just any day in May, but specifically the 1st because I can even pinpoint the exact date that I stopped formally dieting.

That month I was coming through the other side of a horrendous Easter. Not because anyone had been hurt or poorly, no-one had been unhappy or fallen out, not at all, in fact in hindsight it had been a wonderful holiday. But I was blind to it because, yet again, another diet had failed. I had just fallen into an almighty two week binge leaving me at my lowest ever ebb and the guilt was terrible. I was searching Google late into the night for solutions on food addiction and binge-starve eating disorder, buying books on sugar addiction and I was convinced that I had an eating problem so profound that I would be living with it forever.

This probably sounds very dramatic and to look at me at over eleven stone you would never have placed me as having an eating disorder of the traditional kind, but disordered my eating most definitely was. My life was all-consumed by food and the constant control needed around it. I could rattle off at a moment's notice the diet value of anything edible, what category it fitted into, whether it was a high fibre or calcium food and whether it produced a quick weight-loss. I could tell you what I had eaten for every meal for at least the past week and I had a list as long as my arm of foods I avoided because they caused a bad result on the scales.

The omnipresent discipline around food infiltrated everything like some terrible parasite affecting my marriage and children. The number on the scales was an all-consuming obsession and every waking moment held the pressure that I should be doing something to achieve that good result. Even if I had been 'on plan' (a phrase any dieter knows all too well) there was always something I could be doing better. Eat less, avoid carbohydrates, eat courgetti instead of spaghetti, eat fruit instead of yogurt. The list was endless.

I would avoid going places and doing activities or pastimes which would expose me to food. Baking was off the cards unless it was tasteless diet food which my kids took no enjoyment of. No ice cream from the Mr Whippy van for me and no popcorn at the cinema. The suggestion of a coffee and cake from my husband would be met with a thunderous response of 'you know I can't have that' and the ensuing silence as he ate his would be, at best, frosty or we would just avoid it altogether. If my daughter made cupcakes and asked me to have one, I would make up some terrible excuse and watch her little face fall. I would go hungry (and boy would everyone pay for that). On one side I congratulated myself on staying strong, on the other I felt terrible.

Dieting ruled my life and, to look at it from the other side, this all seems insane, but I suspect my story is very similar to many people reading this book. Control was the aim of the game. Absolute and all-consuming control. The problem is, life isn't controllable.

Inevitably would come the day that one off plan mouthful would result in a flip in behaviour of nothing short of alarming proportions. I became a one woman eating machine, bolting down contraband foods until I would feel physically sick. Shopping sprees would ensue where, like a crazy woman, I would go from aisle to aisle filling my basket with cakes, biscuits, crisps and ice cream. I would stop by the coffee shop and buy the biggest, cream-laden drink on the menu with at least two, if not three cakes and the bakery on the way back would yield a multi-pack of cookies and doughnuts. Texts would be sent to my husband announcing that I was 'Off Plan' and boy was I. Like an addict I would eat in the car, hide the wrappers in the bin and smuggle away the evidence. It was a one way track to mental and physical carnage and the guilt and shame that came with it were crippling.

This is where, in May 2019, my journey into the anti-diet movement began. This advocated removing all food restrictions and rules and allowed me to eat whatever I wanted as long as I was listening to my body, following my hunger cues and eating consciously. It all sounded great!

Without a doubt moving away from formal dieting gave me a much better relationship with food. The black and white rules eased into more nuanced guidelines of monitoring how food made me feel, eating mindfully and accepting all foods to be equal. My binges reduced significantly and my diet became more balanced as I ate food groups such as carbohydrates, avocadoes and nuts - all the while marvelling at how I wasn't piling on the weight. This was awesome. I could eat a slice of cake without eating the whole thing and eat a few biscuits without finishing the packet.

As advocated, I listened with fierce concentration to my body's signals and took on a new obsession centring around whether I had eaten correctly and met my body's needs. As with before, this new way of eating came with its own language and so instead of talking about points, macros, syns or calories I was now using the language of honouring my body and health at every size. However, as with dieting, this new set of instructions also came with the ability for me to beat myself up over them. I knew I shouldn't eat quickly or anywhere I was distracted (such as in front of the TV), I needed to obey my hunger and I constantly fixated on whether I had correctly stopped when I was full. The paranoia continued. I had swapped one food-orientated neurosis for another.

Predictably, my eating became increasingly erratic as I failed to perfectly follow these directions and the ensuing guilt grew as I didn't meet the standards. The fact of the matter was - whichever method I was following, if I hadn't eaten according to the directions I had by definition blown it and I was 'off plan' - and what did I turn to comfort, yep you've guessed it, food.

CHAPTER 2

SO WHY DO WE EAT?

This may seem like a daft question as fundamentally we all know why we need to eat. But, in our current culture flooded with weight loss fears, obesity and size zero models food has grown into something much more complex.

Let me spin you a tale, if I may, about how it would be if we treated any other life-essential function (such as breathing or drinking fluids) the way we treat food. If I take, for example, going to the toilet just to demonstrate the excessive level we have now gotten into:

Imagine deciding that you're not happy with your current toilet-going habits and decide that you need to do something about it. Perhaps you discuss this with your friends over a glass of wine or with work colleagues that your toilet-habits are not what they used to be. Perhaps you've seen in a magazine someone who has had amazing success with changing their toilet-going with a certain method and so, filled with enthusiasm, you sign up and go along every week to discuss with others how often and how much you go to the toilet. You keep a toilet-going journal and you review each week your toilet-going habits and pull apart any time where your toilet going wasn't according to plan. Perhaps you then pick up a book that says you can only go to the toilet between 10am and 6pm and to limit the number of times you can go to the toilet in that time. Perhaps you have toilet 'fast' days and days when you can relieve yourself at will. Or perhaps you look into your toilet-going behaviours – did you fully relieve yourself, did you listen to your need to go and were you were fully satisfied with your last trip to the toilet. You search social media to compare yourself to others and try to copy their toilet-going behaviours. I could go on, but I think I've probably painted enough of a picture.

The whole concept would be insane. To take it one step further, try and do this for ten, twenty, thirty or even more years. Anyone doing this would think about going to the toilet *ALL* the time, they would worry about it, talk about it, over-plan, panic about it and over-think it. Worse than that, they would feel *guilt* over it and, tragically, their life would become overtaken by what should be nothing more than a normal bodily function.

My point is, because all these plans put food right at the centre of your mind they, by definition, cause food to take over a disproportionate and obsessively controlling role in your life.

CHAPTER 3

THE FICKLE FRIEND

The fundamental flaw in all this is that food and eating are too imperfect to be so heavily relied upon. The level of perfection required by weight management schemes over a life-essential process is simply just not possible. Worse than that, striving for it will do nothing more than shred every ounce of self-belief you have until your entire self-confidence ends up being built on this imperfect foundation.

There will always be somewhere you could have tried harder – did I eat too much? Could I have made a better choice? Did I really need that? Did I really eat when I was hungry? Did I stop when I was exactly full? The list is endless, and therefore so is the stick to beat yourself with. There will always be that feeling you could have done better. In short, you'll always feel rubbish about yourself.

Ask any parent or work colleague whether they did perfectly all week? Very few will say 'Oh yes!', because to say that you've achieved absolute perfection in something over such a period of time and with so many factors is nigh on impossible. There will always have been a time when you snapped at someone on the phone, made a mistake at work or lost your patience at a fractious child. Outside influences such as other people and unforeseen problems or personal worries such as emotions, hormones, illness or tiredness all come into play and require a level of control which is nothing short of super-human.

Diets will have us all believe that control and perfection is possible 100% of the time when we accept that this isn't possible in any other walk of life. Food and eating by definition are imperfect and you will never (and I mean never) get it completely right - how many times have you heard your naturally slim friend say 'Oh I ate too much'? Unfortunately the damage this does to our mental wellbeing is catastrophic and very few weight loss methods acknowledge the mental load that striving for constant control has on our psychological wellbeing. Search any weight loss forum however and it is sadly filled with heart-breaking stories of how terrible people feel and how downhearted they are purely because of food.

So, if being off plan is so catastrophic why don't dieters stay on track? On one side it is about restriction – both on what we eat but also on *how* we naturally eat. Think of any child and tell them they can't watch TV or eat quickly and all you'll hear for the next 24 hours is a never-ending monologue of how desperate they are to watch Peppa Pig or how they hate eating so slowly, finding with vicious and exhausting effectiveness a way of talking you round. Then, once they do get hold of that forbidden fruit, you can guarantee a solid twelve hours of chain-watching cartoons or wolfing down food from dawn until dusk. In short, restriction creates the perfect conditions for an unbalanced binge-fast relationship. The parallels between this and that constant, driving need in my head for that prohibited Costa coffee didn't take much to see.

However a second and, I would argue more important, factor is the *emotional* link many people have with food. For anyone who has used the term 'comfort-eating' this may sound light-hearted and kind of obvious but this is part of deeper and much more fundamental link to many people's dysfunctional relationship with eating.

In our complex relationship with food, for many of us it has become something we turn to during times of difficulty, stress or quiet to find our feel-good factor. How many times have you opened that packet of cookies when you have been over your head at work or dived into a family-sized bag of crisps when the kids have gone to bed? In short, we start attaching emotions to food and eating to pick ourselves up is embedded deep within many people's psyche. Unfortunately what can make us feel good can conversely also make us feel bad and in pinning our emotions to food, with every dieting triumph also comes associated feelings of personal failure with every disaster. To pick ourselves up again we turn to, yet again, food. The best way I can show you this is below:

1. Food starts to be used for a feel-good factor or comfort

2. This causes physical changes to our body

3. Food now starts to make us feel bad (cycle repeats as food is used to find comfort, or continues to below)

4. An element of control is introduced to consumption and/or eating behaviours associating how we eat with feelings of personal achievement

5. Standards of perfection and over-thinking of food leads to 'off plan' binges

6. Food and eating associated with feelings of personal failure, guilt and low self-esteem

7. Cycle repeats as food is used to find comfort or feel-good factor

Thinking back, I can tell you exactly where I started to use food to get my feel good factor, and (ahem) it was a long time ago. I moved from living abroad to the UK and I started being bullied at school. I have the most exceptional mum who tried everything she could to make my transition easier however my usual feel-good activities of swimming and playing on the beach disappeared and, instead, I started to get my feel-good factor from eating. My brother, on the other hand, found his pick-me-up in sports which, to this day he still has. You only have to ask my sister-in-law and she will tell you at length that without exercise he becomes grumpy and impossible to live with. Sport is where he gets his feel-good kicks and sense of achievement from where as I found mine in food and eating.

Where this all falls apart is that food is not the natural place to get your sense of achievement or feel-good factor from, it is simply not where it belongs. As touched on at the beginning of the book, food's natural place is as a mechanism for keeping us alive, no different than breathing or drinking. We do not derive our self-achievement from how well we've blinked that day or build up our self-esteem from our exceptional water consumption – the very idea would be ludicrous. By keeping food at the centre of their plans, many dieting and eating regimes continue to fuel this self-fulfilling cycle of guilt and comfort eating, bringing us further and further down with every repetition.

Naturally slim people and children do not engage in this cycle because they simply do not associate food with emotions. I come back to our example of a young child, if you ask them what makes them *feel* good it is unlikely they'll say food. They might *like* food (I know mine certainly do) but when it comes to something which makes them *feel* good they'll probably say playing, seeing their friends, cuddles or watching their favourite film. Eating is something they do, but not something they derive their feelings of achievement or failure from. Likewise, naturally slim people do not show extremes in their eating behaviour because, for them, food holds no element of judgement. They therefore have the ability to normalise their intake of food without overthinking it and so instinctively regulate their weight according to their body's needs.

CHAPTER 4

PUTTING FOOD BACK IN ITS PLACE

So to build a healthier, more balanced relationship with food this emotional attachment needs to be broken and our feel-good vibes need to come from their rightful source - our own personal achievements. By doing this, food can then go back to its natural place as something to enjoy and fuel our bodies.

As I started developing this thinking I began observing the naturally slim people around me and their behaviours, as well as unpicking my own feelings and behaviours around food which I really didn't like. Gradually these developed into five distinct areas:

One Size Doesn't Fit All

The first realisation began as I started to look at those around me. When I thought about my friends or family they weren't all the same - of course they weren't. We each had our own personalities, interests, likes and dislikes. In our day to day lives we actively accept and celebrate this and yet, when it comes to weight loss, we often put all our faith in single models of behaviour believing they'll work for everyone.

Many parents-to-be when they first expect a baby delve into piles of parenting manuals and sources of advice; devouring case studies, top tips and baby timetables at an astonishing rate. In the face of doubting our own ability we naturally search for answers in these hallowed holy grails of knowledge, however no-one tells you that your child is blissfully unaware of these new rules.

'It's not working!' you wail at 2am as their screaming wakes up the entire neighbourhood, they go on hunger strike and develop a temper to rival Vlad the Impaler. Your seemingly perfect child is uncontrollable – they aren't doing anything the book says. 'What am I doing wrong?' you cry and the simple answer is absolutely nothing.

However, ask a parent expecting their second child if they've read any of these books and they'll say 'Nope' because they've learned (probably the hard way) that no child is the same and we naturally work around what is best for each individual. The point is that we are all unique and in any other part of life we would not expect millions of people to follow the same rules and for it to work seamlessly for everyone. In reality we tailor what we do to our own individual needs and that's exactly how we should manage our relationship with food and eating.

Gradually Does It

My second realisation came from an unlikely source - veganism. Late in 2019 I jumped on the idea; I watched 'The Game Changers' and I was convinced. Every single thing I watched or read advocated that such a change in diet should be done over a period time - many people recommending up to a year of gradual adjustments. In typical fashion however I went at it all guns blazing and made the transition in five days - I filled the cupboards with everything vegan, swapped the milk and mayonnaise and every meal was turned on its head. I felt so virtuous I practically had a shiny glowing halo around my head. This was it, I had done it.

Unfortunately I hadn't. It lasted about three weeks until I fell off the wagon with spectacular fashion after eating a pizza with non-vegan cheese on it. That tiny 'off plan' moment was enough to send me spiralling off my newfound lifestyle and I was back to eating meat, dairy and eggs like they were going out of fashion. It didn't take much to see the similarities between this and the black and white parallels in thinking that come with dieting.

More extreme than this, diets turn our lives upside down. There are new rules to follow and slogans to learn, classifications of food to understand and exercises to suddenly take up. The change is massive and although no-one would advocate a swap from meat-eating to a plant based diet overnight we somehow think it is completely possible when taking up a new weight loss regime.

Slow incremental change however is neither popular nor fashionable in the dieting industry. How often have you heard the strap line 'Lose half a stone in two weeks', 'Drop a dress size for summer' or 'Get in that little black dress for Christmas'? Lemon juice, maple syrup and extreme yoga all seem to hold the answer to a quick fix, but they are unmaintainable and every fall from the waggon comes with the same self-flagellation known to every person who's ever tried to lose weight. As I started to think about successful, *sustainable* behavioural change one key factor was clear. It was *gradual* – the sum of small changes built up over time.

Going Steady

Which brings me neatly onto my third area. When delving deep down into what I really hated in my relationship with food the wild binge-fast eating extremes were definitely number one on the list. The strictly and perfectly on plan Dr Jekyll to my ferociously (and often rapidly) off plan Mr Hyde. My self-judgement on food was so black and white that I was always either 100% on plan or, by definition, 100% off plan. There was no room for flexibility in the middle. I can't even imagine what these massive variations in consumption ever did physically to my body (other than gradually accumulated weight gain) but the effect on my mental health was devastating.

In this, I yet again turn to our trusty example child or naturally slim person. To watch them eat they simply don't show such massive excesses in their behaviours with food. They eat what they fancy, sometimes a little too much, sometimes too little, sometimes they skip a meal but, in short, food is not something they overthink or question. Children and naturally slim people instinctively accept the normal ebb and flow of consumption allowing them to be secure and stable in their eating behaviours.

As I questioned my habitually slim husband on this he looked hilariously baffled when I asked him how he *felt* about food because, to him, eating is something he does but which it would never occur to him to critique or hold feelings over. If I was to build a sustainable relationship with food, I realised I needed to break these high expectations of perfection and instead see food as something which has inherent flexibility with steadiness at the core rather than the need for precision.

The Feel Good Factor

This is a fundamental theme and which is deeply rooted in what follows in the rest of this book. As I've mentioned before, no-one likes to beat themselves up more than a dieter and, to look at any weight loss chat room or forum it is sadly clear how many people have such tragically low self-esteem and personal perceptions of failure. It is important to remember that food guilt is not something we're born with and, to return to our example child, they generally have a high overall sense of self-achievement and reward. Think of how a child glows when you tell them they've done a great job and how they accept and embrace this, they fill themselves up with how good it feels and often endeavour to repeat the experience.

As I began this journey of observation I realised that generally when I'm feeling good about myself I am naturally prone to eat better. Like that child I engage in a healthier cycle of achievement, feeling good about myself and, in turn, building on this sense of reward through further positive behaviours.

Unfortunately, as dieters, we often place this sense of achievement on our 100% control around food which, as I've explained before, is too complex and prone to failure to be relied upon. Instead of this I realised that if I could build a sense of accomplishment away from food and from another, more dependable, source I could build that sense of achievement and positive cycle on more stable foundations. This would allow my relationship with eating to stabilise as I naturally built my self-esteem and obtained my feel-good factor from elsewhere.

Be Crystal Clear

Now this is a funny one. If building positive behaviours and accomplishments were key to my success I needed to know what I wanted these achievements to be. However when I started thinking about my personal goals they were bizarrely vague. For years (if not decades) I had held myself up to the ideal of 'eating healthier' or 'doing more exercise' but had never actually put any meaning to what I actually meant by these.

If you ask any project manager what they do when they first have a task assigned to them, one of the first things they'll say is that they figure out how to break the larger task into smaller, more manageable assignments. They decide what these are, how they're going to achieve them, what order to tackle them in and when. If any project manager kept their scheme at that high-level task of say, building a football stadium, and left it at that the project would simply never get off the ground.

The great news is that we are all natural project managers. For example, if I said to my husband 'I fancy going on holiday' and left it at that we'd never leave the drive - how could we, it wouldn't mean anything. To make any desire into something we really want we first make decisions on things like what we're going to do, what's realistic, what we need and how we're going to get there. In essence, we'd turn our dreams into a realisable plan of achievable goals.

However, I realised that when it came to my life aspirations I often didn't do this and then berated myself for not reaching these ambiguous goals. So the final key point is this; I needed to take these life-ambitions and make them real by breaking them down into small, definable goals which I <u>knew</u> I could achieve. Step by step I could then take solace in knowing that every time I completed an achievement I was getting closer to what I'd always wanted, and that sounded great.

CHAPTER 5

SO HOW DO WE DO THIS FOR REAL?

This is the point where I wouldn't blame you for thinking this all sounds great in theory, but if you're anything like me you may have tried many times before to make changes or to break your emotional attachment to food and ended up right back where you started. Here I'm going to reassure you that it really is simple and you'll be pleased to hear it doesn't involve a single food rule to learn or journal to keep. It's not even *about* food or eating, instead it's about relocating your emotions and sense of achievement right back where they belong – in your successes.

Now, if you're anything like me in my dieting days my response would have been 'but I have no successes'. And I feel you – bear with me.

Taking you back to our cycle of emotionally-driven eating; by relocating your self-achievement away from food this vitally removes the life-support system from the demoralising sequence and repetition of 'eating to feel good – guilt from eating – eating to feel good'. Instead we're going to build your sense of achievement away from food and instead from goals personal to you, introducing the much simpler, self-fulfilling cycle below:

1. Setting of an achievable goal

2. Completion of the goal

3. Sense of pride and feel-good factor

4. Growing sense of confidence and self-esteem

5. Desire for further feel-good factor causes cycle to repeat

The first, and *only*, thing I'm going to ask you to do therefore is to think of one goal, *one* small achievable action that you *know* you can accomplish over the next seven days. That's all.

Making Your Goal

When thinking about your goal set the bar low, and I mean very low. Choose a goal which will make you feel really good about yourself and which could be part of your big over-arching life-dreams or could be something completely standalone. Whatever it is it must be something absolutely personal to you and which *you* want to achieve.

As you begin to formulate your goal there has to be no shred of doubt in your head that you can fulfil it, even on your busiest or most chaotic of days. If you have even the slightest niggling concern that something might stop you or that it feels too much then it probably is and it's worth rethinking.

Purely to give you an example, as I started on my journey my very first goal was to do ten minutes of hula-hooping per day. Even as a busy working mum I knew that, without a doubt, I could always find ten minutes and this fed directly into my bigger life-achievement of wanting to do more exercise. It was a really good place to start and, with the bar set low, I knew that as soon as I had completed those ten minutes I had achieved my aim and I could focus every ounce of my feel-good factor on it – even if everything else in my day was going to pot I still felt really proud of myself.

To give you an idea of what other goals could look like there are some examples below, or you may already have one of your own in mind:

- Eat one piece of fruit a day

- Go for a fifteen minute walk three times a week

- Read a bedtime story with your child every night

- Drink one glass of water per day

- Complete fifteen minutes of a language course three times a week

Choosing your own specific goal is something which I simply cannot decide for you and where this method fundamentally differs from any other one-size-fits-all. Your goal will be based deep within your personal aspirations of what you want and what you want to change, what you enjoy and what will feel great to you.

Ask yourself what you'd *really* like to work towards or change and what you could do as a simple first step. You might have lots of ideas or may be finding it difficult to think of a goal – don't worry. If you are struggling to bring together your thoughts or to formulate a goal try jotting down some ideas on a piece of paper or start with those high-rise dreams of what you'd like to achieve and start breaking them down smaller and smaller until they become something achievable that you can put into action.

Making It Clearer

As you'll see from the examples above, each one is specific rather than; 'I'll eat more fruit', 'I'll go for a walk' or 'I'll learn a new language'. As your ideas start to develop choose just one and start to make it specific – a single, defined task with an associated time. Your goal doesn't have to be daily, although I do encourage it be frequent enough to be constantly building on that essential sense of achievement and also, here I beg you, make it realistic. It is better to set your goal low and over-achieve than too high and fall by the wayside. If there is any part of you that feels that knot of hesitation that it might not be manageable or that something will get in the way, then realign. You have to know that you can do it and not even a herd of wild horses will get in your way.

If your goal isn't about food or exercise, don't worry, in fact I strongly advocate that as you build on your goals (which I'll come to later) you develop a range of achievements which feed into your feel-good factor. Because eating healthily and exercise were high on my list of life-ambitions my first goals just happened to be in this area, however as time went on they became part of a much wider, holistic package. The one thing I would caution is to avoid making negative or restrictive goals such as 'I won't drink Coke' or 'I'll only eat wholemeal bread'. This sets you up to reinstate those constraints and rules of perfection which are so hard to maintain. Try instead to nudge yourself towards the positive behaviours you *want* to incorporate such as 'I'll drink one glass of water every day' or 'I'll have wholemeal bread for lunch' to create a more positive move and mind-set.

This brings me onto the final part of developing your aim. It *has* to be in your control and this is why I would never advocate specific weekly weight losses as a goal. The result on the scales is affected by many factors – water retention, hormones, illness, what you've recently eaten or drunk to name but a few. An exact loss on the scales holds no guarantee and puts restriction and negative objectives right in the centre of your aspirations. The most innocent 'I'll stay on plan all week' translates to a very pressurised 24/7 stint of perfection with an extra level of restriction, overthinking of food, questioning whether you could have done better and guilt on the side. The goal (although seemingly simple) is actually huge and so complex it is, at best, exhausting at worst going to catastrophically fail – along with your self-esteem. Instead, try to implement a regular activity in which you are in absolute personal control. Once this is completed you can then hand yourself your metaphorical gold star and feel that grin spread across your face as big as a Cheshire Cat.

CHAPTER 6

WHAT HAPPENS NOW?

So, have you got your aim for the next seven days? Is it realistic and in your control? If you have, then brilliant! If you haven't, don't worry, keep reading and give yourself some time to think and develop one that will work for you. It will come in time and may involve a little trial and error as you work it out.

The First Seven Days

It really now is as simple as putting your new-found goal into action. Whatever it may be, the aim is to turn your ambition into a daily activity. Be aware that, in this newfound excitement, it is easy for that familiar competitive urge to drive you to push harder or to up the stakes. At times like this I would strongly encourage you to reign yourself back in and remind yourself of your original goal and stick to it. If you came up with lots of ideas you may even be tempted to introduce two, three or maybe even more and here I am going to add a note of caution - remember my rush for the vegan finish line and how unsustainable dramatic change is. The aim is for small, gradual adjustments that build up over time. However tempting it may be to go for gold, for now just stick to one goal and your chance will come to build in time.

You may equally find that, as you transition away from the dieting mind-set, negative self-talk may still try and chip away at your successes, talking them down as small or insignificant. When compared with the almighty overhaul that diets require it is easy for your goals to seem small-fry and trivial. If you do have a moment like this, feel empowered that you are making sustainable changes at your own pace and on your own terms. If you find a goal, such as an exercise class, is pushing you beyond your own enjoyment, feel happy to step back and acknowledge that it is not right for you - that's completely ok. Remember that the ability for steadiness in your goals is key and that great successes come from stable on-going change rather than a massive undertaking which is then abandoned after a few weeks.

Make sure to acknowledge and celebrate your achievements. You're doing an incredible thing which will improve your health and wellbeing for years to come. I highly recommend you develop the most focused tunnel vision, zoning in on the goal you are fulfilling and how each one is getting you closer to where you want to be. Feel great every time you complete your goal - even to the point of giving yourself a metaphorical (or physical) gold star. Fill yourself with the excitement of these changes and the improvements you are actively making to your life - you really are amazing.

After The First Week

As I've hinted, once you've completed the first seven days this is now your chance to begin building on your goal. Yet again this is something I can only guide you with as it will be completely and utterly personal to you. If, and only if you feel ready, add in a second goal to implement along with your first for the following seven days. This second aim should follow the same principles as your first; that it is small, manageable and absolutely within your control. It might build on, or into, your first goal (for example increasing the length of time), or it might be something completely different. If you feel happy with where you are right now and don't feel the need to add anything new, that's great. What's important is what feels right and manageable for you right now.

Week by week you now follow the same process of adding new goals or changing existing ones every seven days, and at your own pace, until you reach a steady plateau you are comfortable with. In your first month I would encourage you to add no more than one goal per week to make sure that new-starter eagerness does not balloon into something overwhelming and unmanageable. Instead, aim to settle into a gentle stride of sustained and positive change; starting new goals, building on existing ones, changing or adapting old ones or even ditching any that don't feel right for you. Nothing about this is set in stone.

As you become more relaxed into the process you'll probably find your own natural pace of change and discover that the addition and changing of goals becomes more fluid as you naturally build your achievements into everyday life.

You may have long periods where no new goals are set or conversely times when you want to build in something new. Illness or injury may result in goals being realigned to put caring for yourself first, or holidays may need simpler goals which you can easily fit into your day. You may even find that as you tune into your body you begin to introduce actions purely because they feel good and what started as goals evolve into everyday behaviours that you want to do without thinking. The aim is not to drive yourself harder and harder so that by the end of the year you have a list of fifty-two things to do every day but to settle into a happy status quo and healthy balance of change that feels great to you.

CHAPTER 7

SO WHERE DOES FOOD COME IN THIS?

You may be asking at this point where food and eating come into this and the good news is that, by focusing your emotions and sense of achievement within your goals, food now becomes something which holds stability and the steadiness at the core and returns to its natural function as something to fuel your body.

Dieting and the Scales

As you start to build and focus on your goals eating now morphs into something which you do and enjoy but without emotion or judgement attached to it. There are two possible routes you can take for eating: you can either follow a diet of your choice or eat according to your body's cues. The joy of this is that there are no wrong answers and no one-size-fits all. Although I acknowledge that dieting has its danger areas I also realise that food plans and the scales provide a framework and reassurance for many. The good thing is that it is entirely up to each individual to know what will work best for them.

If continuing on an eating plan feels right for you then setting goals to increase your self-esteem and introduce positive self-achievements will only do great things in helping to support you. As you build in this new healthier way of life keep in mind how important it is that food finds its natural and proportionate place and be aware of how your diet may be influencing this. Dieting, by its nature, can throw the balance of thinking about food out of kilter but it is more than possible to continue on an eating plan and protect yourself as long as you put some consideration into how you can manage any potentially negative effects.

Firstly I would encourage you to cultivate an awareness of any damaging impacts an eating plan may be having on your feelings of accomplishment. Remember that diets promote a rapid pace of change and by being hyper-aware of this message you can protect yourself from any feelings of doubt or uncertainty that this might create. Remember that sustainable change, although this may be slower, is key to your long term success. With this in mind, there is absolutely no reason why your goals cannot be something which supports you in your diet plan but be wary of being caught up in the drive to make them too ambitious to meet the need for results.

To protect yourself from the wild swings of on plan/off plan eating behaviour keep at the centre of your mind that perfection with food is simply not possible and to remove any expectations of flawlessness or associated self-judgement. Instead try to work to accept flexibility in your eating and reiterate that a sustained change of 90% all of the time is better than 100% perfection only some of the time and the aim is for steadiness and stability.

As I've cautioned before, in order to protect your goals, avoid weekly aims with a specific weight loss target and instead focus on achievements that are actively in your control. If at any point anxieties about food start to grow in your head, shift your focus strongly and decisively to your feel-good achievements and what great things you're doing to improve your health and wellbeing. Employ that tunnel-vision and fill yourself up with pride and congratulate yourself on what a difference you're making – you're doing great.

The same mentality for dieting also applies to the scales; many naturally slim people do not weigh themselves on a daily or weekly basis however I recognise that the scales are a source of reassurance for many people, especially when trying a new way of life. If weighing yourself regularly is something you wish to continue then great and you know what works best for you. The same as with dieting, in order to protect your sense of self-esteem and achievement I would encourage you to be hyper-aware of how that number can affect your motivation and behaviours – especially if the result is not what you hoped for.

Exactly as with food, put some thought into how you will keep the number on the scales in perspective to all the good you are doing. It is very easy when regularly weighing yourself to wholly pin your measures of success on weight loss and therefore a disappointing result can bring the perception of all your successes to come crashing down.

If the number on the scales does begin to overwhelm you, employ the same tactics as with dieting of fiercely focusing on your achievements and imagine where your new goals will take you in three, six or even twelve months' time. Celebrate changes in your body as much as any change on the scales: do your clothes fit better? Do your limbs move more easily? Can you climb the stairs without being out of breath? Build a way of seeing your body and health through many positive and different perspectives rather than just your weight. Allow for flexibility in your body as it naturally fluctuates and adapts, remembering that the aim is for holistic long term change rather than for drastic crash dieting.

If you feel that either dieting, weighing yourself or both have a negative influence on you and your relationship with food then moving to a way of eating which tunes into your body is the second option outlined below.

What If I Want To Stop Dieting

It is one of the greatest ironies that torments many slimmers that they battle away eating celery and cabbage soup while their naturally slim friends seem to eat loads and never diet. Tuning into their bodies and meeting their hunger needs is how many naturally slim people effortlessly eat and subconsciously manage their weight whilst tucking into everything from tangerines to tiramisu.

It could be from the outset that you feel you want to move away from dieting or, as your behaviours change and you develop a healthier more balanced way of life that you don't feel the need for an eating plan any more. Either way, if dieting or food rules aren't working for you or are making food into a disproportionately overwhelming factor in your life you may feel that a transition towards eating in a way which feels right for you to be a positive move.

The great news is that contrary to what I certainly believed when dieting, moving away from rules is actually really simple. Your body is an incredibly intelligent organism and knows how much food it needs to survive - just like it knows how much air to breathe or times to blink. We consciously do (and can be in control of) many of our life-essential functions, but naturally leave it up to our bodies to lead the way. Just as with any other process, eating is an instinct we all naturally possess – we just need to follow the signals.

The first thing to do is to start listening to your body and for the natural cues that show you your body is in need of food. Again, these will be different for every person – it could be a rumbling stomach, light-headedness or even a change in mood. Don't worry about reaching a prescribed point at which to eat, go with what your body's telling you. An equivalent feeling would be if you needed to visit the bathroom, it wouldn't matter whether you were hopping from leg to leg or just feeling that niggling need to go – either way you would recognise it is time to find a rest room.

If you're feeling hungry and ready for food, eat. Don't worry about over-questioning this or getting it exactly right, let your body lead the way rather than constructing ideals of perfection – you simply won't meet them. When you do feel hungry, go with what you fancy eating. Many people worry that if they do this they'll exist on a diet of white bread, crisps and chocolate but remember that using food to satisfy your hunger is very different from the guilt ridden binges used to pacify emotions. By using your achievements to firmly house your feelings elsewhere this allows you to build a sustainable relationship with food based on feeding your body and satisfying its needs.

When you do get your food, eat it in a way which feels enjoyable and natural to you. Naturally slim people eat in all manners of ways; fast, slow, standing up, in front of the TV, at the table to name but a few. As with hunger, don't overthink it but go with what feels right for you. Go for the bits on your plate that you really fancy first allowing you to enjoy your food and stop when you're done rather than ploughing on past fullness for those tasty bits at the end. Let hunger and your body be the guide and remember that it doesn't matter whether you clear your plate or have unfinished food left over. Although no-one likes waste, as you become more attuned to your appetite you'll find that you naturally plate your portions more and more closely to your needs and that there will be fewer leftovers.

Once you feel about done clear away and move on with your day. Again, don't feel the pressure to pinpoint the exact point of fullness or eating exactly right – there's no such thing. Be aware of what you're eating and how full you're feeling, but there's no need to obsess over it. If you manage to get in the ball-park of feeling satisfied then you're doing brilliantly. Remember that naturally slim people and children show flexibility in how and what they eat and, as we've said before, innately accept the ebb and flow either side of hunger and fullness.

As you learn to follow your body, over time you'll build more and more confidence and assurance and soon fall into a natural way of eating to meet your body's needs supported by your feel-good goals into a holistically healthier way of life.

CHAPTER 8

GOING LONG

I sincerely hope you're full of motivation and excitement to get going – I know I was, and this is the point where I give you the important wider understanding to take this forward as a sustainable, long-term change in your life.

How this process looks will be different for everyone and each person's rate of change will match what is right for them. As unpopular and unfashionable as this is, I'm not selling a quick fix and I acknowledge that patience and avoiding comparisons are not something which sits easily in our society. Unfortunately we are flooded with weight loss media and it is all too easy to compare ourselves to perfectly poised Instagram models, food judgement or drastic weight loss stories and it is easy for these to sow seeds of doubt in our minds. If you do have times like this, ground yourself with the core beliefs of steady and stable behavioural change over time based on achievements which are right for you and remember how these will add up.

There will be wobbly times - it would be wrong of me to promise you there won't be as the most important thing for me to do right now is to equip you for those feelings if they do arise. Remember that even the happiest person in the world has their ups and downs and that these feelings are often short-lived and temporary. There may be times when you have overeaten and experience those nagging feelings of guilt or perhaps your figure isn't changing as fast as you would like. I can almost guarantee that there will be times when you want the change to be faster and it is easy to fall into old habits of picking yourself apart in the mirror or feeling the temptation to give up. Remember that fluctuations in your body on a daily basis are completely normal and that our bodies are incredibly complex living beings. Although adjustments may take a little time to show, just like our nails growing or an injury healing, just because we do not see these changes happening day to day it doesn't mean they aren't happening in the background.

If you do have a down day I strongly encourage you to draw on that pincer-like vision you've practised before and zone in on all those amazing goals you are achieving and what you are accomplishing. Feel that wonderful internal pride fill you up and acknowledge how far you've come. Celebrate changes in your body and think of where the accumulation of all your goals will take you.

As you build a healthier, more stable relationship with food your slim weight will come as you build on your positive behaviours. In a way, observing weight loss as a side effect of this newfound lifestyle, rather than as the aim fundamentally shifts the heat away from the race for a certain number and more as an outcome of your more healthy way of life. As you settle into this more balanced routine take ideas and inspiration from what appeals to you and what excites or feels like it would work for you, however avoid the trap of trying to copy someone else's journey or result – there's simply no faster way to ruin your own self-motivation. You are achieving your own victories and, most importantly, in your own way and have trust that you are doing amazing things – you really are.

CHAPTER 9

ONE LAST NOTE FROM ME

I sincerely hope you have found this book as enjoyable to read as it has been from me to write. It creates a huge amount of hope in me that spreading this message will help as many people as possible to release themselves from impossibly high standards of eating and emotional attachment to food and, in turn, find self-belief, achievement and confidence in themselves.

We are somehow conditioned in our society not to accept praise from either external or internal sources, and so here I am going to take the opportunity to remind you that you are an amazing human being and hopefully you now have the ability to see all the good you do and the incredible achievements you accomplish every day. If this book has helped you to make your goals a reality and, step by step, take you closer towards your aspirations then I feel very privileged to have played even a small part in that.

My one last request is, if you have found this book helpful to not keep it a secret. Let's face it the more people we have who feel happier about themselves and who are bringing positive change to their lives the better. Please spread the word, not only for people struggling with their relationship with food, but also for those in need of increasing their self-esteem – we all deserve to feel amazing about ourselves.

I can't wait to hear your successes and your journeys and wishing you every health and happiness,

Kerry

Find me on the web:

Instagram: feelgoodweightloss_forlife
Facebook: Feel Good Weight Loss for Life

Twitter: @KJohnson_Feelgd

CHAPTER 10

QUESTIONS?

I want to stop weighing myself very regularly, how do I do this?

Again, this is all about what feels right for you. Some people will never want to weigh themselves again and would prefer to rely on their clothes and internal sense of how they're feeling, others will want to flexibly check in from time to time and some regularly (but less often) weigh themselves. This is all about what works for you and there may be a little trial and error in finding the right balance. The one and only thing I would encourage is that the number on the scales is kept in perspective and used as information alongside all the other health benefits and changes in your body you are achieving rather than a single, all-consuming, measure of success.

I'm really struggling, I feel like this is making no difference

Firstly, take a deep breath and take some reassurance that feeling like this is completely normal. It is an old, however unpopular, adage that change takes time and this can be frustrating - we would all love to wake up the next morning and have everything exactly as we dream it to be. We're conditioned to expect (and want) fast results and sometimes things that take time can feel like they're not working. Reassure yourself that your body is altering and, although we can't always see these changes day by day, in the long run they will come to fruition and you'll start to see the noticeable differences from your new, healthier behaviours.

I still want to eat uncontrollably or indulge in unhealthy foods

Again, take a deep breath and reassure yourself that 100% perfection in food is neither expected nor possible. If severe restriction is causing you to over-think food and creating the need to binge then try taking some of the pressure off yourself. Again, I come back to the word steadiness, it is better to have a sustainable and consistent relationship with food than demand perfection only to then binge in response. Try including some of the foods you're craving, enjoy them and then move on with your day focusing your thoughts strongly on your achievements and how good they make you feel.

If you're using food to find comfort, just having this awareness is a huge first step because you now have the ability to turn to what genuinely does make you feel good - your achievements. Again, if you really fancy a certain food, have it and move on with your day without guilt or the need to overthink it. Alternatively you may find you don't fancy it any more. As your relationship with food evolves and health becomes your focus you'll find that you're more and more comfortable with accepting all foods into your diet as something to enjoy as part of a healthy balanced relationship with food and eating.

My feel-good factor from my goals seems to be waning

As you settle into this new way of life and your new goals become more like every-day behaviours it can seem like the shine of these achievements can fade a little. Remember that no goal is set in stone and if you want to shake things up then go for it! Maybe swap to a different exercise or try incorporating a new activity, build on an existing goal or introduce a new one to bring a fresh sense of achievement. Alternatively if an aim really isn't working for you then it may feel right to drop it. Naturally slim people are always trying new things to keep that feeling of interest and challenge alive - let's face it, eating the same meal or watching the same TV programme every day would get pretty dull - so shaking things up is a great step if you want to feel that new sense of success again.

My doctor says I've got to follow certain guidelines for my health

First and foremost your health is what comes first and following the advice of your health professionals is top of that list. There is a nuanced, but important, difference between the motivation to do something because you've been told to and because you *want* to and the latter often comes with a greater internal drive and incentive. Think of how you can turn your health advice into positive goals which mean something and will feel like achievements for you. Perhaps you've been told to limit sugar or take more exercise - these can easily be turned into positive personal goals taking you *towards* behaviours you want to include rather than thinking about restricting what you can't. An example could be to eat two portions of vegetables a day or taking a fifteen minute walk and building up from there to goals which make *you* feel better and meet your health needs.

I think I've done really well but then my smartwatch or phone gives a really disappointing result. It's really affecting my motivation.

We are surrounded by media and gadgets which can provide incredible amounts of information about what we're doing, but which also have the ability to get us down if we haven't generated certain numbers. Remember that your goals are personal *to you* and what makes you *feel* good rather than the drive to achieve certain figures. Feel comfortable in knowing that you are achieving your own personal and sustainable steps to health and at your own pace. Treat these pieces of equipment as just that, fantastic sources of technology which provide information on how many amazing things you *have* achieved (rather than comparing yourself to what you haven't) and celebrate them.

I'm going on holiday - what should I do about my goals?

It would be very familiar to think 'I'll just stop all my goals whilst I'm away and start again when I get back' and how similar this is to the dieting on/off waggon. Although your goals provide lots of benefits in themselves, the vital lifeblood of why they are so important is that they provide your all-important feel-good factor. Without this, there is always the possibility of returning to the original source of feeling good - food, and restarting the 'eating - guilt - eating' cycle again.

With this in mind, I come back to how you decided your original goals - at their core was that they were achievable and completely personal to you. If you are going on holiday, keeping tapped into that feel-good factor is just as important as at any other time and the great thing about your goals are that they hold at their core flexibility and what works for you. When thinking about your holiday, simply re-think to a new goal or goals which you know you can achieve and which will make you feel great. It could be to visit a local site, going for a 10 minute swim or to drink one glass of water for example. Keep any goals super simple, knowing that by maintaining these small achievements whilst you are away you will keep that sense of achievement and return feeling fantastic about yourself.

I'm ill/injured and can't achieve my goals. What do I do?

Firstly, look after yourself. It is vitally important that you do not see this process as a short term battle to push harder, no matter how your body is feeling. What is most important is to look after your health and give your body what it needs. If you're struggling with the thought of not achieving your usual goals, re-align to new ones which focus on meeting your body's needs for rest and recuperation. Allow yourself time to recover and also allow that you may need a period afterwards to build back up to the level of goals you may have been at before. Be patient with your body and give it time - every step in the right direction, no matter how small, is all on the road to success.

I've started a goal with a new activity or new food and I hate it. What do I do, I really don't want to continue.

Then absolutely don't! Goals are 100% personal to you and at their core is flexibility and what feels right for you – if you aren't enjoying a goal then change it, adapt it or ditch it completely until you find something which really does work for you and has you singing from the rooftops on how great it makes you feel.

I'm trying to eat according to my hunger, but at my certain meal time (family dinner time, lunch hour, breakfast before leaving the house etc.) I'm not very hungry. What do I do?

Firstly don't overthink or worry about it. Hunger is not an exact science and modern life means we don't always have the ability to wait until the exact moment of hunger to eat. Approach it exactly as a naturally slim person would, if this is your window to have food then eat to a point that feels good to you and move on. This may mean you eat a little less at that moment - and may eat a little more later. If you're really not hungry you might just want to skip the meal altogether and eat when you're next able to. First and foremost, work with what you can, don't overthink it and carry on with your day.